Editions Péridot 2020

Stop hemorrhoids, anal fissures and constipation

A real, accurate and detailed testimony

first edition

Lise Desjardins

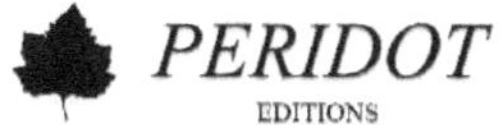

PERIDOT EDITIONS

Table of content

Dedication

I dedicate this little book to you, my dear readers, as well as to all the people around you who suffer from constipation, hemorrhoids and annal fissures. Trust your healing ability.

I wish you all the best. Be blessed.

Lise Desjardins

Warning

This book is not a prescription and is not based on any diagnosis. It is only a question of sharing my journey by retracing the advice in matters of hygiene of life and health which I was given. No product is recommended. Those who helped me are not drugs, but natural foods or supplements. It would be simplistic if my personal story were transposed to that of the reader.

In any case, this text can in no way substitute for medical diagnosis and replace the medicines prescribed by your doctor. Consult quickly. No need to be overly modest or shy. The medical profession has seen much worse.

It seems essential to me to warn you that chronic constipation is not harmless and can in some cases be a symptom of a more serious illness requiring emergency hospital care (intestinal obstruction for example).

It is therefore essential to speak to trusted doctors and health practitioners taking the time to listen to you and carry out all the necessary examinations and health analyzes or to call the emergency services if necessary.

Similarly, internal hemorrhoidal disease can be complicated by a thrombosed prolapse which is a real emergency.

Consult !

Introduction

Why I wrote a book on constipation, anal fissures and hemorrhoids even while I'm not a doctor ?

I have seen around me that many people suffering from chronic constipation, hemorrhoids and anal fissures, despite the different remedies: " home ", advised in the media or by different doctors.

Having suffered from this problem myself, I know how much it can ruin everyday life. That's why I share here how I managed to completely overcome the problem of constipation, anal fissures and no longer suffer from my hemorrhoids without surgery.

Of course all bodies are different, have their own stories and it is up to each of us to make our own path to a better health.

An old story

I suffered from my first hemorrhoid at the age of 22 following my first and last half-marathon. The pain (mild, I understood it later) lasted a few days and dissipated concomitantly with taking a cream treatment (with carraghenate, Titanium dioxide, zinc oxide).

Very episodically the pain returned and was always relieved by the famous ointment it seems, that I had obtained myself in pharmacy without consulting a doctor. The subject seemed too embarrassing for me. I was not totally ignorant of the matter, my father and my grandmother suffering from the same problem.

At the time, my lifestyle allowed me to be in an Olympian form with a diet close to macrobiotics (lots of whole grains, legumes, soy, fish and fruit) respected to the letter and more 20 hours of sport per week characterized by cardio (long distance running, athletic strength including a significant amount of deadlifts, squats, bench presses, press, etc.).

Following a life event, I stopped the sport and lost eight kilos and found myself at the limit of healthy weight. My entry into the world of work did not help. I couldn't gain weight.

I can't remember exactly when I started to suffer from chronic constipation, I must have been 28 years old. I remember long business trips with need to eat out, long days to conduct analyzes seated on computer, stress related to my professional career and a personal life complicated.

I'm talking about chronic constipation. Rather, it was to speak very hard droppings, lumpy, an abnormally high circumference, very difficult to expulse, and characterized the morning by a particularly hard cap and wide.

I suffered a lot in the bathroom, and what had to happen has happened: one day on a business trip, I pushed so hard to free myself that I caused two anal fissures.

I started with a long, very long, too long period of self-medication with my cream (with carraghenate, Titanium dioxide, zinc oxide).

No matter how much I ate vegetables, nothing helped. The stools remained very hard interspersed with diarrhea no less painful at defecation.

I consulted my general practitioner sporadically who suggested an osmotic laxative and another type of cream. She then tried different kind of laxatives and cream and proposed me taking psyllium. Psyllium seemed to have and effect firstly but did not persist.

I hardly ate any more, usually soups, green vegetables, muesli and cheese. Nothing helped.

As I was taking a lot of osmotic laxative in self-medication, I disrupted my stomach, with acid lifts that prevented from sleeping and irritated my throat, ruining my voice of opera singer.

My GP was prescribed different treatments with proton pump inhibitors which I tested alternately. I was reduced to consult a gastroenterologist - proctologist.

After anoscopy, a fibroscopy gastric and a biopsy, the diagnosis fell:

- hemorrhoids accompanied with two anal fissures,

- wide opening of the pylore and the cardia, bile reflux, probably bile gastritis but no Helicobacter pylori.

The gastroenterologist sentenced me to surgery and my general practitioner to treatment with proton pump inhibitors for life.

I could not resign myself to surgery, given my difficulty already healing from my anal fissures, my unresolved constipation and the prospect of a long and painful recovery and random success.

Furthermore, I could not resign myself so young to the continuous taking of medical treatment, even if these options are suitable for many people.

In my entourage, I have a motor disabled person successfully operated on for prolapse or even people taking proton pump inhibitors without problem and for whom the situation is well suited.

At the same time, I sprained my spine while diving into the pool.

Under the advice of my general practitioner, I consulted an osteopath.

Unfortunately, he could do nothing for me compared to my back. However, I took advantage of the meeting to tell him about my problems digestion.

He manipulated me for three sessions the stomach. Concomitantly. I also took a herbal tea against acid reflux under the advice of my voice teacher at the herbalism in Place Clichy in Paris (The main ingredient was licorice with also agar agar and other plants - beware the liquorice is dangerous in case of hyper tension). You can call them if you have any question.

Meanwhile, I thought my stomach problems was not arranged by the collapse of my back linked to a sedentary lifestyle and I was the effort to sit up advantage.

Without being able to determine whether it was these treatments that helped me heal from my acid / bile lifts or my body's return to normal, the fact is that I was much better. The pains woke up very sporadically under strong stress. If in doubt, I had took 1 or 2 tablets of proton pump inhibitors under these circumstances (Lanzoprasol). The pain was gone.

I was eating only green beans, I was drinkink only prune juice, nothing worked. The pain in the bathroom was excruciating. Sometimes constipation was alternated with diarrhea. This did not prevent the suffering, even if in this case it was less.

One day asking for yet another can of laxatives osmotic in a pharmacy, a pharmacist suggested that I take probiotics kept in the refrigerator, in this case Ergyphilus Comfort Intestinal Balance© from Nutergia laboratories.

I was immediately much better, with significantly improved droppings. However, the pain at the defecation, although less severe, was still there.

I periodically resumed boxes of Ergyphilus when constipation was returned (for example following an anti-biotic treatment following an infection of the gums).

During a hiring medical examination in a new position, I met a listening occupational doctor with whom I spoke about my problems. She advised me to take a fund treatment, including Léoderm Santé© based on Omega 3, Evening Primrose oil, vitamin C, PP and B8 as well as Piasclédine© with avocado and soybean oil to promote healing of my anal fissures. I completed the cocktail with fish oil.

After few months, I was better but I was still in pain.

Point noticeable, the skin of my face, dry and rough had become more gentle.

Following a personal motivation seminar, I trained to get in touch with people I did not know.

I was on a train trip and next to me sat a young woman reading literature on hygiene. I finished by talk to her and she indicated me that she was studying naturopathy in order to change of job.

She explained to me how much naturopathy had changed her life and that of those around her. She told me that I had to try.

I chose an inspiring name on the phone book of a naturopath also a pharmacy phd and made an appointment.

Following an in-depth study of my case, the naturopath provides me with:

- general recommendations,

- a specific detoxification treatment.

I returned 3 months later again for final recommendations.

Il you need personnal advice, you can take an appointement with this naturopath.

Appointment are possible by Skype, FaceTime, WhatsApp, teleconsultation doctolib if need on the website bellow :

The general recommendations

Dietary recommendations

You may already be aware of these tips or some of these general tips. I confess I didn't know everything. In particular I did'nt know it was necessary to avoid abusing cereals. I thought that 's muesli and granola was good for health, that is not the case for every body!

- Avoid the abuse of cereals, and if you must eat them, soak them for a few hours before cooking them (in "new" water).

- Avoid white flour and gluten (wheat, barley, oats, rye, spelled): pasta, white bread... Avoid white rice.

- Use whole or semi-complete cereals (even flour, rice, pasta and bread, pie dough, etc.), ancestral wheats (small spelled or khamut) and gluten-free (quinoa, buckwheat, millet, amaranth , wholegrain rice, lupine…)

- Avoid bad fats (saturated and trans): frying, margarine, palm oil, pastries, crisps, red meat, cold meats…

- Use polyunsaturated vegetable fats rich in:

> Omega 3 from plants: oil organic first cold pressed camelina, canola, flaxseed, walnuts,

hemp, perilla to keep in refrigerator (they favrose blood circulation and make their flexibility to cell membranes).

Omega 3 from animals: small fatty fish (sardines, herring, mackerel, occasionally salmon, tuna, etc.).

Omega 6: safflower oil, bourache, evening primrose, pumpkin seeds…

Omega 9: olive oil, black olives, oilseeds (almonds, walnuts, hazelnuts, cashews, pumpkin seeds, flax, sunflower, sesame...)

- Avoid dairy products, especially cows dairy products: yogurt, milk, cream, butter and cheese… (preferably eat fresh sheep / goat cheese with raw milk, unpasteurized if possible in your country, once every 15 days).

- No soy in any forms (tofu, yogurt, milk).

- Increase the consumption of fresh seasonal fruits and vegetables (abundant source of vitamins, antioxidants, minerals, fibers). They can be frozen if needed, but avoid preserves. The preferred foods are cooked green vegetables (steamed), basifying vegetables (pumpkin, sweet potato, etc.), ripe or stewed fresh fruit (except stewed citrus), red fruit (flavonoids) and soaked dried fruit (prunes, figs). Avoid raw vegetables for a while. Eat citrus, spinach, parsley and tomatoes, rich in vitamin C.

- Fruits should be taken outside of meals: 30 minutes before or at least 3 hours after a meal. It is possible to eat fruits and vegetables together, in the absence of cereals and animal products.

- Be careful with vegetable proteins such as lentils. They can be irritating to the intestines. Consume in small quantities and always with cooked vegetables.

- Favor as much as possible cooking at gentle steam, which does not affect the vitamins and minerals. Avoid high temperature cooking (for preventing cancer) and avoid the microwave.

- The diet should if possible be organic and seasonal (or without treatment after harvest), avoid aliments distorted by industry (refining, colorants, preservatives, flavors, sugar added). Think to look at the ingredients. We are happy in France to have a strong regulation for that.

- Drink enough (at least eight glasses a day). It is absolutely essential! If possible, drink a flat weakly mineralized water under 100 mg/L of dry residue (suitable for the preparation of bottles of infants). This kind of water is better for kidneys

- Foods to avoid are chili, pepper, gravy dishes, chocolate.

- Go to the bathroom when the need be felt.
- Do not stay a long time in the bathroom, because the thrust force dilates the veins and promotes the onset of the crisis.
- Try to defecate in the equivalent of a squatting position, for example in a chamber pot. Other solutions exist such as the use by any means of a step/a stool. Just raise the knees so that they are - above the hips and the bust is well leaning forward. You can also sit crouched for a few moments before going to the bathroom.
- Avoid rubbing too hard by wiping yourself after the saddle. Use water compresses, a shower or a bidet.

Other recommendations

Do not wear tight clothes, day or night (panties, pants of course but also any other tight clothing on other parts of the body). I know it's fashionable but it's bad for blood circulation.

Use a specific donut cushion for hemorrhoids. At work, if you're annoyed, explain that you broke your tailbone

First specific detoxification treatment

The detoxification treatment was the first essential step in the treatment. The goal was to cleanse the liver. Indeed, the veins of the anus drain towards the heart by crossing the liver (master organ of spring). This is involved in all the management of blood mass and must be perfectly functional in order to avoid the mechanisms of venous stasis. An increase in liver volume compresses the vena cava and creates a reflux that promotes the appearance of hemorrhoids (and varicose veins).

The treatment lasted 3 months and resulted in me losing 2 kg. At the start of the diet, I weighed 52.2 kilograms and after that 50.5 kilograms for 1.70m. I remained vigilant to not go below this weight limit corresponding to a BMI already low 17.5 (BMI = weight / height ^{2}).

Food   instructions

The food instructions were very restrictive (in complement of the general recommendations). Especially at the start. I was wondering how I was going to get out of it. I had to prepare my lunch and at the time I never imagined that I could. Today it is a habit that seems obvious to me.

<u>Breakfast:</u>

- No citrus, no fruit juice

- Crushed banana + a teaspoon of linseed or camelina oil + a tablespoon or two of fresh cistus pollen, fresh seasonal fruit or dried fruit and a small handful of oilseeds maximum + if possible 1 tablespoon to camu camu + if possible ½ bunch parsley.

Warning, oilseeds are very tasty but in large quantities, they are very bad for the kidney function. Do not exceed a small handful a day.

Fresh cistus pollen is the richest pollen in lactoferments from the digestive tract of the bee. The micronutrients present in this pollen make it an excellent ally to restore its internal balance in the event of persistent fatigue and / or intestinal disorders. Cistus pollen is naturally rich in vitamins B2 and B3 which contribute to the maintenance of normal mucous membranes, the reduction of fatigue and a normal energy metabolism. In addition, it is also rich in vitamin B9 and source of vitamin B6, iron, zinc, selenium which contribute to the normal functioning of the immune system. This type of pollen can be ordered on the website https://www.pollenergie.fr/ , with the following partner code (75PM02) which will allow you to benefit from a reduction in shipping costs.

Please note fresh cistus pollen must be kept in the freezer upon receipt. It can then be eaten as it is, coming out of the freezer. This pollen I think has helped me considerably.

<u>At noon:</u>

- Vegetable 60% (steamed)

- Animal protein 30%: fish, eggs, poultry (red meat no more than once a week)

- Starchy food 10%: preferably gluten-free (prefer quinoa, buckwheat, potato, sweet potato, squash, etc.).

- One or two spoon of olive oil and rapeseed (or flax / camelina)oil

- Aromatic herbs: parsley, coriander...

The naturopath insisted that I keep animal proteins because of my weight below the recommendations. If I had been a vegetarian, even greater vigilance would have been required for the diet with appropriate blood monitoring.

<u>Teatime:</u>

-    Fruit including citrus if it is the season.

<u>Dinner:</u>

- Vegetable proteins 10%: lentils, chickpeas, split peas, fresh or dry algae in flakes, mushroom, quinoa, hulled hemp.

- Starchy food: 20%

- Vegetables: 70% - one or two spoons of olive and rapeseed (or flax / camelina)oil

- Aromatic herbs: parsley, coriander...

- Sunflower seeds, pumpkin seeds, sprouted seeds

- Dessert: cooked fruit

In general, food supplements are not to be preferred. The body must theoretically be able to find everything it needs in food. It is however complicated.

On the advice of my naturopath before every meal I drank gel aloe - vera (30 ml in a glass of water, PurAloé© or Aragan© brand for instance). I did not notice any effect, but it is difficult to know if it is this or that ingredient, or such combination of ingredients that contributed to the cure.

Besides, I also took:

- 2 months of Desmodium (Salpan) in parapharmacy, which gave me some belching.

- for 21 days the following supplements (can be purchase by phone on this website https://www.la-royale.com):

> Roy-eau Acido: 2 in the morning (favorable action on the acid-base system)

> Roy-eau Hepa: 2 the evening before the meal (supports the hepatodigestive functions)

Roy-Eau Acido contains 10% of black currant leaves, Java tea Leaves, Pellitory of the Wall, common fumitory, Rosemary, Viola tricolor, elder flower, goldenrod, cherry tails, strawberry leaves.

Roy-eau Hepa contains Linden, Milk thistle, artichoke.

In the morning and outside the meals, drink herbal tea: a mixture of lemon balm, rosemary, thyme.

Lemon balm is particularly useful against stress, insomnia and overwork. It is recognized as antispasmodic, antiviral, digestive and effective against anxiety. People with hemorroides, constipation or annale fissures are often very stressed.

Rosemary has digestive and diuretic properties, and it also helps fight infections.

Thyme has spasmolytic properties. It helps relieve intestinal disturbances such as diarrhea, bloating, flatulence, various colopathies. It is also antiseptic and antifungal.

Physical activity

My revitalization cure would not have been complete without an exercise program, the objective being to sweat to detoxify the body.

The recommendation is to resume physical activity two to three times a week without it being intensive so as not to aggravate the hemorrhoids: outdoor sports in priority, moderate cardiovascular training, especially walking, swimming, supplemented with yoga and Pilates.

Be carefull, I noticed when I had acid lifts that swimming increased it due to a brewing too violent of the stomach (even water aerobics standing).

It has been difficult for me to put physical activity back into my busy schedule, but it is a vital necessity.

I keep in mind the following sentence: "the chair kills", sedentary lifestyle kills.

Dozens of chronic diseases are favored by time spent sitting and physical inactivity: A sedentary lifestyle is one of the risk factors for hemorrhoids. Apart from crises, it is therefore important to practice regular physical activity. This physical activity will facilitate intestinal transit and limit hemorrhoidal attacks and the constipation.

More generally, a sedentary lifestyle increases the risk of cancer by 25%, hypertension, obesity, depression, Alzheimer's disease. The first treatment for these diseases is walking. Neurologists say that brain food is physical activity.

For my part, I try to move throughout the day without making any violent physical effort:

- walking (ideally in Nordic walking with arm movement and if possible sticks),

- movements of Pilates to straighten the back (and thereby relieve pressure on the digestive tract, focusing on exercises carried vertically)

- water aerobics (inutile to take classes, moving in water is sufficient)

- any movement of gym / dance allowing to gently untie the body (in particular dance like "Twist dance" is good for constipation), also to carry out at home every day. It's a funny way to fight constipation.

The purpose of physical activity is to restore circulation in the body on a daily basis.

Be careful in case of a severe hemorrhoidal crisis, it is recommended to ban all physical activity and especially the most violent (especially carrying heavy loads).

In case of pain, abdomino- diaphragmatic breathing (through the belly), legs crossed cross-legged to decongest the small pelvis can help. This is an opportunity for a meditation session.

What seemed to me the most effective in this diet, which I continue today is the change of breakfast with the cessation of muesli.

Yes, for years I ate a good muesli in oat milk. Before going to the naturopath, I already had the feeling that this muesli (very simple with no added sugar bought in organic stores) was a problem. I had started to consume it in porridge (that is to say cooked in water or oat milk), and had noticed a slight reduction in the inconveniences.

Furthermore, an essential point that I never deviate from is taking a sip of oil in the morning. This is what has greatly improved my stools. Indeed the hardness of the stool was largely due to the absence of consumption of good fats it seems.

Second cure to keep in time

Food instructions

<u>Breakfast:</u>

- Same as detoxification programm

- No citrus, no fruit juice

- Crushed banana + a teaspoon of linseed or camelina oil + a tablespoon or two of fresh cistus pollen, fresh seasonal fruit or dried fruit and a small handful of oilseeds maximum + if possible 1 tablespoon of camu camu + if possible ½ bunch parsley.

<u>Noon:</u>

- Vegetable: 50%

- Plant or animal proteins 30%: fish, eggs, poultry (red meat no more than once a week)

- Starchy food 20%: preferably gluten-free (prefer quinoa, buckwheat, potato, sweet potato, squash, etc.)

- 1 or 2 tablespoons of vegetable oil

The naturopath insisted that I keep animal protein because of my weight below the recommendations.

<u>Tea Time:</u>

- Fruit including citrus if it is the season.

- A few seeds / nuts in small quantities.

<u>Dinner:</u>

- 30% starchy food (sweet potato, potato, squash, buckwheat, etc.),

- 10% vegetable proteins (lentils, chickpeas, beans, etc.),

- 60% vegetables,

- 1 or 2 tablespoons of vegetable oil.

<u>Herbal tea:</u>

Rosemary, lemon balm, ginger, blackcurrant leaves, throughout the day for three months and then adapt as needed.

In addition I supplemented this new diet with the following cure available on the site https://www.la-royale.com/ 10 days per month for two months:

- Circulation complex n°1: 2 capsules 3times per day

- Circulation complex n° 2: 2 capsules 3times per day

The circulation complex n°1 corresponds to a box of 200 capsules dosed at:

- 50% sheet vine red (vitis vinifera 125 mg),
- 20% of leaf hamamelis (hamamelis virginiana 50mg),
- 20 % of root fragon (ruscus aculeatus 50 mg)
- and 10% of flowering tops of goldenrod (solidago virgaure 25 mg), in micronized form.

Circulation complex n°2 corresponds to a box of 200 capsules dosed at 250 mg, including:

- 125 mg of horse chestnut (seed),
- 50 mg of Ginkgo biloba (leaf),
- 50 mg of sweet clover (flowering tops)
- and 25 mg viburnum (bark) in micronized form.

Despite a regularized transit with the diet, I still suffered from my hemorrhoids, even if much less. Determined to heal and under the influence of an intuition (for ice), I decided to take things in hand with a cure made up of the following three elements:

- Cream NEO FITOROID BIOPOMMADE endorectal 40ML ABOCA (advised by my naturopath) for two months: This cream contains lyophilized extracts of Helichrysum flowering tops lipophilic fraction (Helydol) and root of Fragon false holly ; gel leaf Aloe Vera dried ; aqueous solution of Helichrysum flowering tops ; Oily extracts of St. John's wort flowering tops ; Jojoba oil; Shea Butter; Essential oils of Melaleuca , Cypress and Peppermint.

- Injection of the following mixture using pipettes:

Peppermint essential oil 2 ml

Cypress essential oil always green 2 ml

Pistachio Lentisk essential oil 1 ml

Inophylated Calophyll vegetable oil 5 ml

Please note, this recipe found in the french magazine "Alternative Santé" is recommended for external use (external application on hemorrhoids) and not internal as I do.

Essential oils can be toxic. For my part I took the personal initiative to inject it internally rectally. The use of this mixture internally is absolutely not recommended without medical advice, essential oils can be dangerous for internal use. This treatment is of course to be prohibited for pregnant women. For my part I injected myself morning and evening the equivalent of 0.25 to 0.5 ml of this mixture for one or two months.

I prepared this mixture myself. It was also possible to ask a pharmacist or an herbalist to do so. I obtained all the ingredients and utensils (bottle, graduated cylinder, polyethylene pipette) from Aroma-zone french website for example.

Peppermint essential oil is particularly analgesic. It calms the itching. It is refreshing. It plays a bactericidal and fungicidal and also anti-inflammatory role (around 3 € 10 ml).

The evergreen cypress essential oil has long been known for its exceptional tonic and circulatory properties (around € 2.50 10 ml).

The essential oil of Lentisk pistachio is traditionally known for its decongestant and circulatory properties (around 10 € 5 ml).

Calophyll vegetable oil is also called "Tamanu ". It is known for its many properties, rare for a vegetable oil: anti-inflammatory, healing, anti-infectious, analgesic, stimulating blood circulation. I love this oil which also helps me a lot for rosacea on my face (around 7 € 100 ml). I found this recipe here on the alternative health website
https://www.alternativesante.fr/circulation/hemorroides
-l-automedication-qui-marche

- Last but not least: the use of ice.

Yes I think the ice cream helped me considerably, for free. Even if that makes my general practitioner smile and even my nathuropath. I kept in my freezer boxes of ice to make very large ice cubes which I put in a basin of water which made it possible to obtain a seat bath below 10 ° C. I stayed as long as I could (i.e. a few minutes at most), sitting in this cold water. I avoided exposing my genitals (not easy for a woman). I also tried the ice suppository and most often at the end of the shower the spraying with cold water. Then I was putting the essential oil mixture.

After two months of this shock treatment, I was relieved, after six years of pain.

Idem detoxification treatment.

It is absolutely essential, by all means, in all weathers.
And of course hydrate yourself.

General conclusion

In conclusion, I would say that this journey required time, good encounters, money. Budgetary arbitrations are necessary to be able to have quality food. People in need should not hesitate to glean in the markets while waiting to improve their finance when possible. Also remember to check whether your mutual insurance reimburses self-medication products and natural medicines. It's better to make these sacrifices than to immediately take the risk of a surgery that presents risks and does not necessarily treat the source of the problem.

Most of the time, your doctor will recommend a laxative and a lidocaine cream (an anesthetic) to relieve your hemorrhoid attacks. But by doing so, you treat the consequence without treating the cause of the problem.

Plant glossary

ARTICHOKE

The artichoke is a domesticated and cultivated thistle. The one we know has existed since the end of the Middle Ages in Europe. It would be a thistle transformed by horticulturalists by selection. It is native to North Africa (Egypt and even Ethiopia) and is said to have been brought to Sicily by the Arabs. The artichoke is a vegetable rich in particular in polyphenols: such as flavonoids but also acid-phenols. Its antioxidant activity would be excellent especially in front of all the other vegetables and also on par with red berries such as cranberries, blackberries or blueberries. The artichoke stock would thus be the vegetable richest in polyphenols in the diet, ahead of parsley as well as Brussels sprouts. The artichoke is known to be hepatoprotective, it would promote digestion and fight against constipation, particularly chronic. The artichoke is also composed of silymarin and flavanolignans. These molecules are said to stimulate the regeneration of liver tissue.

Black haw are shrubs or small trees frequently planted in gardens for the decorative aspect of their flowers, and their fruits often very appreciated by birds. They are used for menstrual pain, prolapse of the uterus, also for heavy periods or morning sickness, menopause disorders. Preventing the risk of miscarriages and nervous accidents during pregnancy, postpartum pain, heavy leg syndrome and of course hemorrhoids can also be treated by Black haw.

Butcher's broom is a species of shrub growing on the Mediterranean rim and in the Atlantic area. The rhizome has circulatory properties. It is indeed a diuretic and vasoconstrictor. This is why it has the nickname "plant of light legs". Also its root has emollient characteristics. It also contains a steroid glycoside called ruscogenin. This is used in ointments for hemorrhoids or dark circles and bags under the eyes.

CALOPHYLLE INOPHYLE

An oil rich in assets and multi-properties

This high quality oil obtained, very rich in pulp and antioxidant active ingredients (vitamin E and polyphenols), sanitizers (inophyllin A) and repairers (Calaustraline and inophyllolide) is used as an ingredient in your preparations. It is an ideal oil for formulating treatments for skin with imperfections, delicate, or for the realization of treatments to fight stretch marks.

Polyphenols that also have tonic activity make it an ideal oil to compose light leg care or fight against facial redness.

From an ethical trade, the oil we offer is virgin, 100% pure and natural, obtained by first cold pressure and certified organic.

CHERRY   TAILS

Cherry Tails are primarily used for their properties of elimination (diuretic and detoxifying) well known but also against inflammation of the urinary tract, cystitis and renal colic. They are also useful for treating overweight, to detoxify the body by promoting the functioning of the kidneys. ☐

CISTUS

Cistus are shrubs growing mainly on the Mediterranean arc. They appreciate dry, with silice but also calcareous and of course sunny soils. They have the distinction of regenerating and even multiplying, especially after frequent fires. They bloom from spring to early summer. Rich in vegetable proteins, fibers, amino acids, vitamins, antioxidants, cistus pollen is rich in essential nutriments. It is notably the pollen richest in lactoferments. It strengthens the intestinal flora, the first natural barrier against external aggressions and, among other things, helps fight constipation.

COMMON FUMITORY, EARTH SMOKE

Common fumitory are plants that flower until mid-summer. They grow in fields, vacant lots and also on the edges of paths. They would have several virtues in particular depurative on the kidneys, the gall bladder and the liver. They would be cholagogue, diuretic, choleretic, tonic and laxative. They are used for difficult digestions, but also in many skin pathologies such as eczema and atopic dermatitis.

CYPRESS ALWAYS GREEN

The essential oil of Cypress always green is known for a long time for its exceptional tonic and circulatory qualities. Regulatory, Cypress essential oil always green is also traditionally known to reduce excessive sweating. Its soothing action makes the essential oil of Cypress always green a must to calm coughing.

ELDER

Elder flowers are traditionally used to facilitate the functions of urinary and digestive elimination. Their "anti-acid " action is linked to their high content of calcium salts.

GINKO BILBOA

The Forty ecus tree or Silver Apricot Tree is a species of tree, the only representative of the Ginkgoaceae family and of the ginkgophyta division. It is a panchronic species because it is the oldest family of trees known. It would have appeared even before the appearance of dinosaurs over 270 million years ago. Ginko is well known in herbal medicine, mainly for its venotonic virtues, but also vasodilatory and neuroprotective. Ginkgo is part of the number of drugs and food supplements available in pharmacies intended to strengthen brain functions, memory and blood circulation.

GOLDENROD

The goldenrod is a genus of flowering plants in the Asteraceae family commonly known as solidages, or sheaves of gold that grows in North America and Europe. Some of these species are reputed to have virtues, especially in kidney diseases. Rich in flavonoids of vitamin P type, the goldenrod is also useful in the treatment of varicose veins and therefore hemorrhoids. As such, it enters into the composition of medical specialties, especially in Germany.

Hamamelis are shrubs with foliage originating in North America, Japan and China. The Amerindians had a traditional use taken up by the western colonists. WHO recognizes the use of witch hazel to treat varicose veins and hemorrhoids as well as bruises, sprains, minor wounds and local inflammations of the skin and mucous membranes. □

HORSE CHESTNUT

Horse chestnut is the seed of the common horse chestnut tree. It is not edible. It is used for its veno-tonic properties, especially in the preparation of venous tonics. This seed should of course not be confused with the edible chestnut, fruit of the chestnut tree.

JAVA TEA / ORTHOSIPHON

Orthosiphon is a genus of plants in the Lamiaceae family sometimes called Java tea because of its Indonesian origin. The leaf and the flower head have diuretic and cholagogical properties (facilitates the elimination of bile).

LEMON BALM

Lemon balm is a perennial herb. It should not be confused with the lemongrass used in Asian cuisine. A plant native to the eastern Mediterranean, lemon balm has spread throughout Antiquity throughout Europe. Lemon balm is most often used for its calming and relaxing properties, useful in cases of stress related to constipation and hemorrhoids. In fact, it regulates the nerve impulse, which has a beneficial action on tachycardia. Also it also reduces spasms of the stomach and colon. Furthermore, these antifungal properties are interesting. In infusion, lemon balm has a mild sedative effect and also promotes perspiration, useful for the elimination of toxins.

LINDEN

Lime tree bark is known for its draining properties. The lime tree stimulates emenctories. It is recommended in the treatment of gallstones. Lime tree is traditionally used to facilitate elimination, kidney and digestive functions.

MELILOTUS

Melilotus are herbaceous plants widely visited by bees, formerly cultivated as fodder. Melilotus is a medicinal plant whose flowers are used for their anti-inflammatory and protective properties of the vascular and anti-spasmodic system. In herbal medicine Melilotus is used in the form of a mother tincture to treat heavy legs, but also hot flashes and of course to combat the undesirable effects of menopause thanks to its fluidifying action on the blood. This makes it an interesting herb for hemorrhoids.

MILK THISTLE, St Mary's thistle

Milk thistle is a large plant, biennial, usually exceeding one meter. Milk thistle is composed of lipids in seeds, but also flavonolignans, flavonoids, sterols, phenolic derivatives of tocopherol and mucilages. The World Health Organization (WHO) recognizes the use of the seeds of this plant for the treatment of hepato- biliary digestive diseases. □

PEPPERMINT

Powerful stimulating and refreshing effects.

PISRACIA LENTISCUS

Traditionally known for its decongestant and circulatory virtues and recommended to promote circulatory comfort and regain a feeling of light legs.

RED VINE

For several centuries, red vine leaves have been used in phytotherapy for their beneficial action on venous disorders. The vines contain multiple tannins, carotene, quercetin, quercitrine, sugars, inosite, acids, choline, tartrates and carotene. It is a plant of first choice for the treatment of hemorrhoids!

ROSEMARY

Rosemary is a shrub of the family Lamiaceae (or Labiatae), pushing in the wild around the Mediterranean, particularly in arid and rocky scrubland on calcareous soils. Rosemary has long been used empirically in herbal medicine. Modern studies show the effects of rosemary on different parts of the body. It is notably choleretic and hepatoprotective. These effects have been shown experimentally. Rosemary therefore activates the digestive functions, in particular the work of the gallbladder.

SALPAN (DESMODIUM)

Salpan is a set of herbaceous tropical plants, shrubs or shrubs. Salpan is recognized as hepatoprotective: it thus increases the resistance of the liver cells, especially in cases of inflammation of toxic or infectious origin, for example due to drug treatment or chemotherapy. It would also be effective against viral hepatitis (of course in combination with drug therapy), particularly at the start of the disease.

STRAWBERRY

Strawberry leaves are traditionally considered as a light astringent and are therefore frequently used in herbal teas for gastrointestinal purposes. Their effect is linked to the presence of tannins. ☐

THYME

As an infusion, thyme is a disinfectant for the digestive tracts, often used for example in combination with sage and rosemary. Thyme relieves, for example, difficult digestions. This too can be used for liver disease. It is known against inflammation of the throat, inflammation of paranasal sinuses, and also against the symptoms of bronchitis and even whooping cough. It can also be used in mouthwash in case of inflammation of the gums and in gargling in case of throat irritation or angina. A plant with many virtues!

VIOLA TRICOLOR (Johnny Jump up)

Viola tricolor is a species of herbaceous plant, common throughout Europe. Viola tricolor has a long history of use in traditional medicine due to its anti-inflammatory properties. It is also useful for the treatment of skin conditions, inflammation of the mucous membranes of the respiratory tract. It has laxative and depurative properties, that is to say that it facilitates digestion and that it improves the function of the organs of elimination, or emunctories like the liver, the gall bladder, the kidney, the bladder the intestines.

Emergency measures in summary

In summary, the emergency measures that I retain in the event of a hemorrhoidal crisis and constipation:

For hemorrhoids:

- no violent physical effort during the hemorrhoidal crisis then resumption of regular activity,
- realization of frozen seats baths by protecting the genitals (painkillers and vaso-constrictors),
- application of the recommendations of feeding of this book (and in particular no spices, chocolate, alcohol), drink water,
- application of the following mixture for hemorrhoids: Essential oil of Peppermint 2 ml Essential oil of Cypress always green (*Cupressus sempervirens*) 2 ml Essential oil of Lentisk pistachio (*Pistacia lentiscus*) 1 ml Vegetable oil of Calophylle inophyle 5 ml subject to medical advice (prohibited for pregnant women).

For constipation:

- immediate intake of highly dosed probiotics, of good quality (kept refrigerated at the pharmacy, ask for advice),

- strict application of the feeding recommendations in this book and drink plenty,

- move as much as possible (twist dance),

- stay a little squatting to favor the arrival of the feces.

In both cases:

- medical consultation to have a precise diagnosis (courage, this is nothing dramatic),

- then application of the minimum dietary and physical exercise recommendations of the detoxification treatment and the second treatment to be kept over time to treat the causes and not only the symptoms, subject to medical advice.

Anal fissures take time to heal. You have to be patient and have the best diet possible to help the body heal.

In all cases it is essential to stay relaxed as much as possible, especially in the bathroom. Stress doesn't help.

I wish you all the best.

Be blessed